THE ANTI-AGING CODE.

The Keys to Enjoying Your

Healthiest and Longest Life.

Dr Frank N. Scott

CONTENTS

INTRODUCTION.

The beginning of adulthood is the beginning of an ongoing and continuous process of natural and biological change called aging. Several body processes start to gradually deteriorate in the early middle years.

At no particular age do people become old or aged. Old age has traditionally been defined as commencing at age 65. But history, not biology, was the cause. The eligible age for Medicare insurance in the United States was set at 65 in 1965. This age is close to when the majority of people in economically developed cultures retire.

Typical Aging.

Individuals frequently question whether their aging-related experiences are normal or pathological. Even though everyone ages somewhat differently, aging itself can cause various changes. So, despite being undesirable, such changes are thought to be normal and are frequently referred to as "pure aging." Any one who lives long enough experiences these changes, and the notion of pure aging includes this universality. The modifications are normal and usually unavoidable. Take for example, the eye's lens becomes thick, stiff, and loses the ability to focus on close objects like reading materials as people age (a disorder called presbyopia).

The changes that come with normal aging increases a person's risk of developing specific illnesses. For instance, tooth loss is more common in older persons. Nonetheless, regular dental visits, a reduced sugar intake, and diligent brushing and flossing may lessen the likelihood of tooth loss. Hence, tooth loss is a preventable aspect of aging even if it is common with age.

Successful (healthy) Aging.

Healthy aging is defined as delaying or reducing the negative impacts of aging. Maintaining both mental and physical wellness, preventing illnesses, and continuing to be active and independent are all aspects of healthy aging. Most people find that as they become older, maintaining overall health involves more work. Creating certain beneficial behaviors, such as

- Maintaining a healthy diet.
- Avoiding excessive alcohol consumption and cigarette smoking.
- Regular exercise.
- Maintaining mental activity.

The earlier one establishes these behaviors, the better. It is, however, never too late to start. People can exert some control over their aging process in this way.

CHAPTER ONE

HOW WE AGE.

Aging is a natural part of life. Given the increased tiredness, weakening bones, and poor health that typically accompanies aging, there is no denying it. Age is, in reality, the main risk factor for a wide range of illnesses, such as Alzheimer's, cancer, cataracts, and macular degeneration. Large knowledge gaps still exist in the aging process itself, even though researchers are making strides in comprehending and managing each of these diseases.

Even at the genetic level, the aging process may be traced back to individual cells, and the age-related die or enters senescence. Senescence is the process by which a cell matures and ceases to divide permanently but does not pass away. In tissues all over the body, a significant proportion of aged (or senescent) cells can accumulate over time. These cells are still active and can emit toxic chemicals that could harm neighboring healthy cells and create inflammation. Cancer and other illnesses could be influenced by senescence.

The development of mutations over time and deficiencies in DNA repair mechanisms are strongly linked to aging symptoms. In actuality, genetic changes in the genes responsible for maintaining our DNA are frequently the root cause of illnesses that result in premature aging. At the molecular level, aging can also be caused by changes in mitochondrial function, a propensity for protein misfolding, and a decline in stem cells' capacity to proliferate.

While many methods, including calorie restriction and genetic modification, have been shown to lengthen the life span in model organisms in the laboratory, these animals may not always be healthier as they age. In the end, aging researchers must discover not just how to prolong life, but also how to stop age-related illnesses and physical decline.

The cellular machinery involved in DNA replication makes errors during the process, changing the DNA sequence. DNA can also be harmed by mutagens such as reactive oxygen species (ROS) or UV radiation. The majority of the time, DNA repair processes restore the damage, but mistakes can persist and mount as organisms age. Moreover, aging has been associated with a decline in DNA repair mechanisms, which makes permanent mistakes more frequent in older animals.

Senescent cells kill themselves or stop reproducing when their DNA has sustained too much damage. Dysfunction and tissue deterioration can result from cell loss. Moreover, senescent cells, despite being essentially dormant, may speed up aging by secreting inflammatory cytokines that are linked to diseases like atherosclerosis and other age-related illnesses. Furthermore, as we age, DNA scaffolding proteins that normally assist in genome stabilization experience changes that affect cell division, senescence, and other aging-related processes.

What Causes Aging? - The Hallmark of Aging.

The mechanisms that contribute to the aging process are hot topics of debate among scientists. Nonetheless, it is generally acknowledged that the functional decrease linked to aging is caused by accumulated damage to genetic information, cells, and tissues that accumulate with age and cannot be restored by the body. It is less apparent, however, what the molecular basis for this harm is and why it can be reversed in young, but not in old, creatures.

Scientists have begun to identify and classify the molecular and cellular hallmarks of aging to better understand the aging process. Nine potential hallmarks are typically thought to be involved in the aging process and work together to define the observable signs of aging. If a similar process deteriorates prematurely and lengthens lifespan while improving health as people age, it is said to be a hallmark of aging.

The Nine Hallmarks of Aging :

1 Genomic instability.

The genome is the entirety of an organism's genetic makeup or DNA.
Almost all the cells in the body have a complete copy of its genome. Every information the body needs to grow and develop is encoded in its genome.
Every one of our body cells, except red blood cells, has the necessary instructions for all cellular operations. Almost 3 billion so-called nucleotides, or individual DNA building pieces, make up human DNA, which serves as the blueprint for each individual's genome.
The appropriate operation of the genome is crucial for the healthy functioning of our body because it carries the instructions for every

function in a cell. Yet, both internal and external factors constantly threaten our genome. UV radiation and air pollution are examples of harmful external impacts. The DNA can be harmed by oxygen radicals created inside the body during respiration. Every single cell in our body experiences up to one million instances every day of DNA damage, according to estimates.

Thankfully, our DNA also carries the instructions for several mechanisms that can recognize and fix such damage. As a result, the genome can be repaired by our cells themselves.

The issue is that these restoration methods are not flawless. Although the majority of DNA damage events can be repaired by our cells, a small percentage of DNA lesions are not correctly restored and are instead encoded as mutations in our genome. These mutations build up over time, especially as we age, and have the potential to negatively affect every element of a cell's function. Individuals who have damaged genome repair mechanisms frequently exhibit symptoms of premature aging. Moreover, DNA damage aids in the growth of cancer.

As said earlier, calorie restriction, or eating less food, has been found to delay the progression of DNA damage over time. Additionally, basic health recommendations like avoiding sunburn, consuming fewer grilled or fried meals, and quitting smoking are all beneficial. This demonstrates that there are strategies to slow down the aging process by lowering DNA damage or enhancing cell repair processes.

2. Telomere Attrition.

Telomere shortening is one type of genomic instability in particular. The human genome's chromosomal ends are known as telomeres. They maintain the stability of our chromosomes and are similar to the sealed end of a shoelace. A chromosome is found in a cell's nucleus. Proteins along with DNA are arranged to form genes on a chromosome. Hence, the chromosome contains proteins and DNA. 23 pairs of chromosomes are present in each cell. The length of the chromosomal ends shortens as humans age because telomeres are shed with each cell division. The cell stops dividing and turns dormant when it reaches a predetermined minimum length. The resulting death or inflammation of such cells might hasten aging and the onset of illnesses.

Telomere shortening is stopped and even reversed by a specialized enzyme known as telomerase. Symptoms of accelerated aging have been seen in mice lacking this enzyme. Therefore, mice with higher telomerase levels have longer lifespans. Telomerase is either hardly or never active in the majority of adult cells. However, because telomerase activity is linked to a variety of cancers, activating it to lengthen life is a risky strategy.

3. Changes in Epigenetics

More than 3 billion nucleotides of the A, T, C, and G kinds make up our genome. The genetic material is tightly wrapped up and packed into the tiny, micrometer-sized nucleus of the cell. The DNA molecule would be 2 meters long if the DNA strand had been unwound and stretched out. In the cell nucleus, histone proteins are encircling the individual DNA strands. Little chemical alterations in both DNA and histones can be utilized to turn specific genes on or off. The epigenome is the result of all these chemical alterations.

During aging, the epigenome changes. Some of the chemical alterations are lost, inserted in the wrong spot, or misplaced. As a result, the regulation of gene activity, or the precise turning on and off of specific genes, also alters. Diet and lifestyle choices have an impact on our epigenome, but so does prolonged stress or certain medications.

4 Loss of Protein Homeostasis.

The instructions for every cellular activity are encoded in the DNA of our cells. Yet, these processes are not carried out by DNA by itself. Instead, our DNA carries instructions for making proteins and enzymes that take over functions and regulate cellular activities. All chemical processes in cells are governed by proteins and enzymes, which also give cells their structure. Proteins must be folded exactly into a very specialized structure, comparable to origami, to perform their functions. The preservation of all proteins' form and abundance is referred to as "protein homeostasis," or simply "proteostasis."

Normal cellular functions cause proteins to become increasingly degraded with age, which also affects how they fold and take on different shapes. Misfolded proteins tend to cluster together, which can be harmful to cells and render them incapable of carrying out their usual functions. For instance, misfolded proteins are the cause of age-related disease Alzheimer's disease.

The cell has several methods to regulate the folding and integrity of proteins due to the significance of maintaining proteostasis. There are methods to both degrade damaged proteins and then build new ones in addition to processes to mend and refold them. For instance, autophagy is a recycling process that can destroy misfolded and damaged proteins. Many research findings point to the significance of proteostasis in aging: The prevalence of misfolded proteins rises with age, and they are linked to several age-related disorders, including Alzheimer's.

5. Uncontrolled Nutrient Sensing

Cells and tissues store energy and expand when nutrients are abundant, and when nutrients are insufficient, mechanisms for balance and repair are triggered. The evolution of this behavior has led to its establishment, and it may be linked to a slowed aging process. The biological processes that detect nutrients become desensitized when cells are repeatedly exposed to excess nutrients, as is the situation with diabetes and obesity. The process that causes cells to improperly react to the signals that typically control energy production, cell development, and other critical cellular activities also takes place during the aging process.

As a result, numerous researchers have looked into how eating habits or how people perceive food affects their aging process. For instance, the insulin signaling pathway is turned off and the longevity of mice increases when the total amount of food consumed is decreased (caloric restriction) or when the organism is made to "think" that it has less food, for instance by the use of certain medicines.

6 Malfunction of the Mitochondria.

A cell needs energy to sustain all cellular functions and chemical activities. The mitochondria are where cells produce their energy. The mitochondria or popularly known as the "powerhouses of the cell" are tiny organelles found inside each cell. They are critical for using the oxygen in our breath to produce energy.

Reactive oxygen species, or ROS, also known as free radicals, are however occasionally created by this mechanism.

Almost every component in a cell, including DNA, proteins, and fatty acids, can be harmed by ROS. There was a time when ROS was believed to be the primary cause of aging. It was once thought that lowering ROS levels would inevitably result in better health and a longer lifespan. Nonetheless, it has long been understood that sometimes having ROS levels reduced has absolutely no impact on health. In certain instances, the situation is even reversed, and a little rise in the amount of ROS within cells has advantageous benefits.

Because of this, it has been determined that ROS in general plays a significant role in signaling cellular stress.

Stress causes cells, tissues, and organs to speed up their maintenance and repair functions. So, the level of ROS must be exactly right—not too much nor too little—for healthy aging.

In general, crucial cellular signaling pathways and functions can be impacted by mitochondrial malfunction. Eventually, the cell's ability to produce energy decreases, and simultaneously, the level of oxidative stress rises, damaging other cellular elements. Hence, mitochondrial failure plays a role in several age-related illnesses, including myopathies and neuropathies.

7 Senescence of cells

Cell division helps an organism expand or allows for the replacement of aged cells in a specific tissue or organ. Yet, this ability eventually wears out since the great majority of cells are unable to divide indefinitely. Senescent cells are those that have stopped replicating permanently. These cells do not, however, perish. Instead, a few of them discharge toxic chemicals into their surroundings, which can injure neighboring cells.

Telomere shortening is one factor in cellular senescence. Yet, there are a variety of other factors, such as DNA damage, that can cause a cell to enter a senescent state.

For several years, it was uncertain whether senescent cells accelerated aging or served as a potent barrier to the growth of cancer. Senescent cells reduced lifespan even in young mice, according to a recent study. Senolytics, or drugs that destroy or silence senescent cells, are now being studied in humans for their potential therapeutic benefits in the treatment of cancer and aging.

8 Stem Cell Fatigue

Our body's tissues and organs must be able to replace worn-out cells and repair damage if we are to maintain overall health. Stem cells, which exist in nearly all tissues, allow our body to regenerate damaged tissues and organs. As stem cells have the potential to divide endlessly and create new cells, they are the primary source of new cells.

When the body or a particular tissue requires new cells, healthy stem cells must have the ability to divide—but only when necessary and under controlled conditions. Age reduces stem cells' capacity to divide, and their capacity to divide just when new cells are required. In the worst-case scenario, the uncontrolled division of the cells leads to cancer.

9 Changes made to intercellular communication

Our body's cells can communicate with one another. Maintaining cell-to-cell contact is essential for our health and affects how quickly we age. Several methods of communication are available to cells. They converse through their physical proximity if they are right next to one another. Yet, it is also feasible to reach cells that are not nearby by releasing specific chemicals. It is even possible to communicate with recipients who are located in entirely different parts of the body by releasing hormones into the bloodstream. This allows various organs to communicate with one another.

In addition to altering the messages cells provide, aging also affects the receiving cells' capacity to react to these signals. Due to the immune system's inability to detect and remove pathogens or defective cells, this dysfunctional communication increases the risk of infections and cancer. Other issues include chronic tissue inflammation.

....

The nine hallmarks of aging unequivocally demonstrate how intricate and flexible the process of aging is at the biological level. The nine hallmarks of aging provide a great foundation for our understanding of the basic biology of aging, even though aging research is continually changing.

In conclusion, aging is not a designed process like development and only evolves as a byproduct; no genes have been created specifically to cause harm and death. This may also be the reason why it varies so much both within and between people.

CHAPTER TWO

PREMATURE AGING

Aging is a drag. We are told it, and as we age, we come to realize it for ourselves. We all strive to maintain our youthful vitality and have an idealized concept of adulthood free from aging in mind. Unfortunately, nature has different intentions.

Every day, we are all engaged in a battle with nature to fend off the symptoms, impacts, and warning signs of aging.

There are billions of dollars worth of items on the market that can help you combat the consequences of aging in whatever way you want, from brain-training mobile games to pills and treatments.

But there is a straightforward rule: The house always wins when you play poker against the casino.

People inevitably age. Our skin, joints, organs, and even memories may start to work less effectively and exhibit indications of deterioration as we age as a result of processes that once occurred properly.

If you're fortunate enough to make it to 100 or beyond, you'll notice this every day as you walk more slowly, recover more slowly, and experience the groaning and straining of once-effortless muscles and joints.

And the majority of people who survive beyond 100 are content to tolerate the adverse effects to experience those latter years.

Premature aging, however, is not covered by the agreement. The abrupt emergence of those signs in your 40s or even 30s can leave you feeling particularly dejected because experiencing these things early was not part of the plan.

Yet, you don't necessarily have to embrace premature aging. Understanding the causes, signs, and therapies for premature aging can give you back control, allow you to postpone the onset of your symptoms to a time when they are more tolerable, or perhaps prevent them completely.

The Symptoms of Early Aging.

The symptoms of accelerated aging are similar to those of normal aging, as you might expect. They simply occur earlier than anticipated.

Signs of aging include things like sunspots, wrinkles, hair loss, and early graying. The effectiveness of your body's production of vital proteins like collagen, hormones like DHT, and mechanisms like cellular regeneration and repair have changed, which is the main cause of all of these issues.

Your body can make the proper proteins and regulate the appropriate responses when you're younger and everything is functioning normally.

Aged Skin

Your skin won't age since it has healthy repair and hydration processes, preventing it from getting thin and haggard. Together with proper cellular turnover, it will also keep healing acute UV damage.

But with time, several events may lead to a slowdown in collagen formation and chemical degradation. As this occurs, things that previously occurred seldom, like sun spots, wrinkles, and inflammation, start to multiply and get worse.

The thinning and loss of hair.

Male pattern baldness, which is medically referred to as androgenic alopecia, is brought on by several factors, but the main one is the excess production of the hormone dihydrotestosterone (DHT), which can significantly the process of regrowing hair follicles and makes those that are currently growing to appear weaker and thinner.

Yet premature hair loss can start as early as a man's adolescent years, and it's frequent among men in their 50s.

Reasons for Premature Aging.

You may look older than you are due to several different circumstances. They fall into a few categories, such as lifestyle, environmental, and hereditary influences.

Environmental Elements.

Several environmental elements can harm, stress, and ultimately trigger early aging indications in your skin. Acne and other aging symptoms are brought on by factors such as facial skin stretching from sleeping inappropriately, sunshine, and air pollution.

But sunshine can be the most important environmental component by a wide margin. Your skin is battered by sunlight, which depletes your Vitamin C reserves. Because vitamin C functions as the body's main antioxidant in the battle against free radicals brought on by UV rays, it is essential for maintaining your health.

Without the capabilities to combat the free radicals produced by radiation, which can prevent your skin cells from replicating correctly or at the right frequency, low levels of vitamin C leave your skin defenseless.

Polluted air, which can rest on your skin and demolish antioxidant reserves in the same way, can cause the same damage.

Lifestyle elements.

Premature aging can be caused by certain lifestyle decisions and habits, such as drinking and smoking, which harm the skin and put additional strain on the body's natural regeneration mechanisms. According to studies, smoking's harmful impacts on skin health can lead to premature aging, delayed wound healing, psoriasis, cancer, and hair loss, among other problems.

A poor diet and not drinking enough water can deprive cells and tissues of the nutrients and supplies they require.

Hydration is necessary for almost all routine biological processes, and skin health is no exception.

Research has linked a lack of water intake to defective dermis tissue, including everything from inflammation to the early aging process.

Genetic Roots.

Extreme cases of premature aging can result from certain genetic conditions, also known as progerin conditions. These are the kinds of conditions that are brought on by genetically induced DNA damage and cell line mutations.

They can shorten a person's lifespan to around 20 years or cause aging process symptoms to appear at puberty. They can also cause symptoms to appear as early as birth. Nuclear proteins that aid in proper cell division, maintenance, and repair is crucial to your body's healthy, youthful appearance. When these proteins are genetically weakened, your tissues, skin, and other organs will exhibit the same signs of aging that typically come from years of natural deterioration.

Werner syndrome and Hutchinson-Gilford syndrome are two well-known instances, despite how uncommon they are.

However, there are therapies to take into account for as many causes as there are for you to exhibit premature aging symptoms.

It's vital to see a doctor right once if you or your children have one of these problems because genetic conditions may need a variety of treatments, and only a small portion of the symptoms of unusual aging conditions can currently be properly addressed.

Other causes, however, can be handled with a range of topicals, vitamins, and dietary adjustments. It comes down to three main strategies: reducing oxidative stress, replacing critical nutrients in the skin tissue and other organs, and effectively treating the symptoms.

Skin

To address all of these vulnerabilities, several therapies are required for the skin, which requires love, care, nutrition, and protection.

The following actions can help prevent premature skin aging:

Consume a Large Amount of water: Water is the foundation of healthy skin and the essence of moisture. It has been demonstrated that drinking more water has a favorable effect on skin effectiveness and quality, particularly in people who consume less water daily.
Even while it is insufficient on its own, it will support other treatments and is important for everything else your body does.
Skin cleaning: Using a cleanser as part of your skincare regimen can help reduce the negative effects of environmental toxins by eliminating them before they cause harm.
Basic face cream can serve as a barrier to block them out in the first place should you wish to take preventative measures.
Stop smoking: Certainly, it could be more challenging than it seems, but there are tools at your disposal to support you as you make this crucial decision for the health of your skin.

Exfoliate: No, really. Exfoliating can help your body reduce lines and wrinkles by introducing newly developed cells at the surface and is an easy way to combat the early signs of aging. It can also remove dull, dead skin cells.

Moreover, think about using a chemical exfoliator, such as a vitamin A compound (also known as a retinoid), which will have the extra anti-aging effect of promoting quicker regeneration.

CHAPTER THREE.

EFFECTS OF AGING ON BODY SYSTEM AND WHAT YOU CAN DO.

You are aware that wrinkles and gray hair are side effects of aging. But do you also know how aging impacts your teeth, heart, and even sexuality? Learn about the changes that come with aging and how to maintain excellent health at any age.

Your Heart and Blood Vessels.

What's going on?

The hardening of the blood vessels and arteries, which makes your heart work harder to pump blood through them, is the most frequent change in the cardiovascular system. To cope with the increasing workload, the cardiac muscles adapt. Your heart rate will remain the same when you're at rest, but it won't increase as it used to when you're exercising. These modifications raise the danger of hypertension and other cardiovascular issues.

What You Can Do.
To encourage heart wellness:
Include some exercise into your everyday regimen: Try out some hobbies you like, like swimming or walking. You can keep your weight under control and reduce your risk of heart disease by engaging in regular, moderate physical activity.
Adopt a balanced diet: Choose lean sources of protein, such as fish, whole grains, fiber-rich foods, and fruits, veggies, and vegetables. Limit salty and foods high in saturated fat.
Avoid smoking: Smoking makes your arteries harder, raises blood pressure, and quickens your heartbeat. If you smoke, it is better to stop earlier while you're still young than later. The dangers of smoking increase with age.

Stress management: Your heart may suffer as a result of stress. Consider taking stress-reduction measures, such as talking therapy, exercise, or meditation.

Obtain adequate rest: Your heart and blood vessels can recover and be repaired with the help of a good night's sleep. Ensure you sleep at least seven to nine hours every night.

Your Muscles, Joints, and Bones
What's going on?

As a person gets older, the bones get weaker and the risk of obtaining a fractured bone increases due to the reduction in the size and density of the bone. You may even grow a little bit shorter. Muscles lose their strength, endurance, and flexibility, which might compromise your stability, balance and coordination.

What You Can Do.

To improve bones, joints, and muscles:

Ensure you are getting enough calcium: The National Academies of Science, Engineering, and Medicine suggests individuals consume at least 1,000 mg of calcium each day. For men and women who are 71 years of age or older, the dosage is increased to 1,200 mg per day. Calcium can be found in dairy products, broccoli, kale, salmon, and tofu, among other foods. Talk to your doctor concerning calcium supplements if you have trouble getting enough calcium from your diet.

Ensure you are getting enough vitamin D: For adults under the age of 70, the daily recommended consumption of vitamin D is 600 international units, while for adults over 70, it is 800 IU. Sunlight is a common source of enough vitamin D for many people. Eggs, milk enriched with vitamin D, tuna, salmon, and vitamin D pills are other sources.

Include some exercise into your everyday regimen: Exercises that place weight on your body, such as walking, running, tennis, stair climbing, and weightlifting, can strengthen your bones and prevent bone loss.

Do not overuse drugs: Avoid smoking, and consume alcohol in moderation. Inquire with your doctor about the recommended daily alcohol intake for your age, sex, and overall health.

Gastrointestinal System.
What's going on?
Older adults may experience increased constipation as a result of structural changes brought on by aging in the large intestine. Lack of exercise, insufficient hydration, and a low-fiber diet are other risk factors. Constipation may also be caused by drugs, such as diuretics and iron supplements, and medical diseases, such as diabetes.

What You Can Do.
Constipation prevention:

Adopt a balanced diet: Make sure to eat plenty of whole grains, fruits, and vegetables as well as other high-fiber foods. Avoid eating too many high-fat meats, dairy items, and sweets as these may make you constipated. Take in plenty of liquids, especially water.

Include some exercise into your everyday regimen: Regular exercise can aid in preventing constipation.

The impulse to urinate shouldn't be resisted. Constipation can result from holding back a bowel movement for too long.

Your Urinary System and Bladder.
What's going on?

As you age, your bladder's elasticity may decrease, necessitating more frequent urination. Weakening of the pelvic floor muscles and bladder muscles may make it challenging for you to empty your bladder or result in you losing bladder management/control (urinary incontinence). Incontinence and difficulty with urinating are two other symptoms of an enlarged or inflammatory prostate in males.

Being overweight, diabetes-related nerve damage, some medications, and alcohol or caffeine usage are additional causes of incontinence.

What You Can Do.

To encourage urinary tract and bladder health:

Visit the bathroom frequently: Think about going to the bathroom regularly, perhaps once every hour. Increase the intervals between your toilet visits gradually.

Keep a healthy weight: Try to maintain a healthy weight or reduce your weight if you're overweight. Overweight can be the leading cause of many health issues.

Avoid smoking: Ask your doctor for assistance in quitting if you smoke or use other tobacco products.

Do some Kegel Exercise: Squeeze the muscles you would use to stop passing gas to exercise your pelvic floor (Kegel exercises). Do it for three seconds at a time, then take a break for three seconds. Repeat the exercise 10 to 12 times in a row. Do three sets every day.

Abstain from bladder irritants: Alcohol, caffeine, acidic foods, carbonated beverages, and acidic foods can exacerbate incontinence.

Avoid constipation: Consume extra fiber and take further measures to prevent constipation, which can make incontinence worse.

Your Capacity for Memory and Thought.

What's going on?

As you become older, your brain experiences changes that could have a little negative impact on your memory or cognitive abilities. Healthy older persons may, for instance, forget familiar names or words or have more trouble multitasking.

What You Can Do.

These actions will help to promote cognitive health:

Include some exercise into your everyday regimen: Your whole body is supplied with more blood during exercise, including your brain. According to studies, regular exercise enhances memory and improves brain health by lowering stress and depression.

Adopt a balanced diet: Your brain may benefit from a heart-healthy diet. Emphasize whole grains, veggies, and fruits. Choose low-fat protein options including fish, lean beef, and skinless chicken. Alcoholism can cause memory loss and confusion.

Keep your mind engaged: Your memory and cognitive abilities may last longer if you maintain your mental activity. You may read, engage in word games, start a new hobby, enroll in classes, or pick up a musical instrument.

Be Social: The prevention of depression and stress, both of which can impede memory, is facilitated by social engagement. You might spend time with family and friends, volunteer at a nearby nonprofit or school, or go to social gatherings.

Give up smoking: If you smoke, giving it up could improve your cognitive function.

See your doctor if you're worried about the loss of memory or other changes in your cognitive abilities.

Your Eyes and Ears.

What's going on?

It becomes more challenging to focus on near objects as you get older. You could become more susceptible to glare and struggle to adjust to various degrees of light. The lens of your eye might become clouded as you age and may impair your vision (cataracts).

Your hearing may also deteriorate. In a busy setting, it may be challenging to hear high frequencies or follow a discussion.

What You Can Do.

To enhance eye and ear health:

Plan frequent medical visits: Regarding glasses, contacts, hearing aids, and other corrective devices, heed the advice of your doctor.

Take safety measures: When you're outside, wear sunglasses or a hat with a wide brim, and when you're near loud machinery or other loud noises, use earplugs.

Your Dental Health.

What's going on?

The gums around your teeth may start to pull away. A dry mouth can also be a side effect of some drugs, including those used to treat allergies, asthma, high blood pressure, and high cholesterol. Your teeth and gums could thus become a little bit more susceptible to decay and infection.

What You Can Do.

To advance dental health:

Brush and floss: Use normal dental floss or interdental brushes to clean between your teeth after brushing twice a day.

Plan frequent medical visits: Regular dental checks should be scheduled with your dentist or dental hygienist.

Your Skin

What's going on?

Your skin thins and loses elasticity and becomes more fragile as you age. Additionally, the fatty tissue just beneath the skin shrinks. If your oil production of your skin reduces, the skin gets drier. It is more likely to have wrinkles and age spots.

What You Can Do.

To encourage glowing skin:

Be gentle with your skin: Use warm, not hot, water to bathe or take a shower. Apply moisturizer and mild soap.

Take safety measures: Use protective clothing and sunscreen whenever you are outside. Regularly check your skin, and let your doctor know if anything changes.

Quit smoking: The importance of quitting smoking as you age can not be overemphasized as it has been repeated severally in this chapter. Smoking causes skin damage, including wrinkles and it can also cause respiratory problems.

Your Weight.

What's going on?

As you get older, the metabolism of your body slows down. You will put on weight if your activity levels decline as you age but your eating habits remain unchanged. Be active and follow a nutritious diet to keep your weight in check.

What You Can Do.

To keep a healthy weight:

Include some exercise into your everyday regimen: You can maintain a healthy weight by engaging in regular, moderate physical activity. You do not have to engage in intense, simply trekking a long distance, jogging, or doing house chores will do just fine. Anything that keeps you physically active.

Adopt a balanced diet: Choose lean sources of protein, such as fish, whole grains, fiber-rich foods, and fruits, veggies, and vegetables. Avoid food with high sugar and saturated fat.

Observe portion sizes: Watch your portion sizes to reduce your calorie intake. It is necessary to take in low calories as you age. High calories can cause many health issues as you age.

Your Sexuality.

What's going on?

Sexual performance and needs may alter with age. You may not be able to enjoy sex if you are ill or on medication. Vaginal dryness in women can make intercourse uncomfortable. Impotence in men may cause them to worry. Erections might not be as solid as they once were, and they might take longer to achieve.

What You Can Do.

To improve your sexual well-being:

Talk to your partner about your needs and worries: You might decide that physical intimacy without sexual activity is best for you, or you might try out various sexual behaviors. You do not have to completely stop having sex as you age. Experiment, be youthful, try out new methods, and be open to learning.

Exercise frequently: Exercise enhances cardiovascular health, flexibility, mood, and self-image, all of which are aspects that contribute to healthy sexual health.

Consult your physician: Your doctor may recommend a specific course of treatment, such as estrogen cream for dry vaginas or oral medication for male erectile dysfunction.

. . . .

It is impossible to stop aging, although certain changes can be made to improve your chances of living a healthy life and spending time with family. Aging is inevitable but your lifestyle and diet can make the process a little less hectic.

If you make deliberate efforts to stay active and to be mindful of the food and the portion you consume you will most likely not need to worry about the deteriorating effects of aging.

It is very possible to age and still be healthy. In the following chapters, we will discuss this food and lifestyle that can be used to promote healthy aging.

CHAPTER FOUR

FOOD FOR HEALTHY AGING.

It is crucial to eat healthy at any age but it becomes more crucial as you age towards midlife. Eating healthy can help you maintain a happy outlook and emotional stability in addition to maintaining your physical health. But, eating healthy doesn't always require sacrifice and dieting. Instead, the emphasis should be on savoring healthful, flavorful cuisine while dining with friends and family.

It's never too late to modify your diet and enhance your mental and emotional well-being, regardless of your age or past eating habits. By changing your diet now, you can:

Enjoy a stronger, longer life: Proper nutrition helps increase immunity, combat chemicals that cause disease, maintain a healthy weight, and lower the chance of heart disease, stroke, hypertension, type-2 diabetes, thinning of the bones, and cancer. A balanced diet, in addition to physical activity, can support increased mobility as you age.

Improve/Sharpen your mind: Consuming fruit, green vegetables, seafood, and nuts rich in omega-3 fatty acids may help people concentrate better and reduce their risk of developing Alzheimer's disease. As you age, green tea's antioxidant content may help to improve memory and mental acuity.

Improved Mood: Healthy meals can increase your energy and improve your appearance, which will improve your attitude and self-esteem. When your body feels well, you are happier both inside and out, therefore everything is connected.

Healthy Eating is More Than Just Food.

It takes more than simply high-quality and diverse cuisine to eat well as you get older. Also, sharing a meal boosts the enjoyment of eating. Dining with others might be just as crucial to your diet as including vitamins. A social setting can help you maintain your meal plan while stimulating your thoughts and making meals more enjoyable.

Healthy meals can be more enjoyable even if you live alone by:

Going on Shopping with Friends or Family: You can catch up on your tasks without getting behind by going shopping with a companion. Also, it's a terrific method to exchange fresh recipe ideas and take advantage of promo sales.

Cooking With Friends or Family: Bring a friend over to share culinary duties; one might make the main course and the other the desert, for instance. Sharing expenses can make cooking with others more affordable for both of you, and it can be a pleasant way to strengthen your connections.

Fostering Social Interaction at Mealtimes: Talking to a friend or loved one at the dinner table can be a significant factor in reducing stress and improving mood. Regularly get the family together and keep informed about everyone's lives. Embrace a friend, coworker, or nearby neighbor.

How to plan A Nutritious Diet for Aging.

Focusing on whole, minimally processed foods that are as close to their natural forms as possible is the secret to healthy eating as your body ages. Finding a healthy diet that is most effective for you may require some trial and error because our bodies react to various foods in different ways based on heredity and other health concerns. Here are some suggestions:

Consume a lot of Fruit and Veggies: Get out of the apple and banana rut by choosing colorful foods instead, such as berries or melons. When it comes to vegetables, select dark, leafy greens that are high in antioxidants, such as kale, spinach, and broccoli, as well as vibrant vegetables like carrots. Vegetables can be made more enticing by adding goat cheese, frying them with garlic or chili flakes, or drizzling them with olive oil.

Choose calcium for strong bones: To avoid osteoporosis and bone fractures, managing bone health as you age requires introducing enough calcium into your system. Milk, yogurt, and cheese, as well as non-dairy options including tofu, broccoli, walnuts, and kale, are also good sources. Learn more here:

Not "no fat," but "good fat": Instead of trying to eliminate fat from your diet, concentrate on consuming healthy fats, such as omega-3s, which help shield your body from disease and improve your mood and cognitive performance.

Change up your protein sources: Consuming adequate high-quality protein can help you think more clearly, raise your stress tolerance, anxiety, and depression, and improve your mood as you become older. However, consuming an excessive amount of protein from meat items like hot dogs, bacon, and salami may make you more susceptible to cancer, heart disease, and other illnesses. Increase your intake of fish, beans, eggs, almonds, and seeds to diversify your protein sources and avoid relying just on red meat.

Consume more fiber: Dietary fiber has several benefits outside of just keeping your body regular. It promotes weight loss, improves the health of your skin, and reduces your risk of diabetes, heart disease, and stroke. It's crucial to get adequate fiber in your diet as your digestion gets less effective as you age. Men over 50 should strive to consume at least 30 grams of fiber daily, while women over 50 should aim for at least 21 grams. Regrettably, the majority of us only receive half of those sums.

Be smart with your choice of carbohydrates: To get more nutrients and fiber while reducing your intake of sugar and refined carbohydrates, choose whole grains rather than processed white flour. While our ability to taste and smell changes as we age, we can still tell sweet flavors apart for the longest, many elderly people consume more sugar and processed carbs than is good. Contrary to complex carbohydrates that are high in fiber, processed or simple carbohydrates (such as white rice, white flour, and refined sugar) can cause a sharp rise in blood sugar followed by a swift drop in blood sugar, leaving you feeling hungry and likely to overeat.

Vital Nutrients and Vitamins As You Age

Water: Your sense of thirst may become less acute as you become older, making you more likely to become dehydrated. Keep in mind to drink water frequently to prevent urinary tract infection, constipation, and even disorientation.

Vitamin B: At the age of 50, your stomach secretes less gastric acid, making it more difficult to absorb vitamin B-12, which is essential for maintaining the health of your blood and neurons. Use fortified foods or vitamin supplements to get the 2.4 mcg of B12 that is advised for daily consumption.

Vitamin D: If you're obese or you get little sun exposure, or if you're older and your skin is less effective at producing vitamin D, talk to your doctor about adding fortified foods or a multivitamin to your diet.

Physical Changes That May Impact Your Nutrition.

Metabolism: Our metabolism decreases every year after the age of 40, and we frequently become less active. To prevent weight gain, it is even more crucial to develop healthy eating and exercise habits.

Diminished senses: You might be tempted to salt your food more heavily than you used to, although older adults require less salt than younger people. This is because older adults tend to lose their sensitivity to salty and bitter tastes first. Instead of using salt to season meals, use healthful oils like olive oil, herbs, and spices.

Medicines and disease: Certain medical conditions or medications can impair taste or appetite, which can again cause older persons to ingest excessive amounts of salt or sugar.

Digestion: As you age, your digestive system slows, producing less saliva and stomach acid, which makes it harder for your body to consume certain vitamins and minerals like B12, B6, and folic acid, which are essential to preserving mental clarity and healthy circulation. Increase your fiber intake and discuss potential supplements with your doctor.

Malnutrition.

Malnutrition is a serious health concern that affects older persons and is brought on by undereating, inadequate nutritional intake, and aging-related intestinal issues. Fatigue, sadness, a weakened immune system, anemia, weakness, and digestive, lung, and cardiac issues are all brought on by malnutrition.

To avoid malnutrition as you get older:

- Take in nutrient-rich foods.
- Make tasty meals accessible.
- Between meals, take snacks.
- Eat as much of the time as you can with the company.
- Enlist assistance in food preparation.

Eating Properly As You Age

The greatest thing you can do to improve your health as you age is to eat a balanced diet. As you get older, eating healthfully can help you avoid several health issues like cardiovascular disease, stroke, diabetes, and obesity. Also, it might prevent certain ailments from growing worse. Maintaining a nutritious diet that complements any medication you may be taking is crucial for people aging with disabilities.

But what is a healthy diet? Dietary advice can occasionally be complex or intimidating. You might use these suggestions to assess your eating habits and identify any healthy modifications.

- When you have a balanced diet, you can occasionally indulge in your favorite processed foods or sweets as long as your diet overall consists of a range of fresh, wholesome foods. Read the nutrition labels on processed goods you purchase, and aim to reduce your intake of:

- Substances like fructose or corn syrup, which are present in many packaged snack items, are examples of added sugars. Men should have no more added sugar than 9 teaspoons daily, while women should consume no more than 6 teaspoons.

- Trans fats, also referred to as partially hydrogenated oils are additives used to extend the shelf life of some processed foods.

- Calcium - A small amount of salt is acceptable, but consuming more than 2,300 milligrams of sodium per day (about a teaspoon) is not advised. Foods in cans, frozen dinners, and snacks like potato chips sometimes have high salt content.

- Limiting saturated fats, which are present in meat, cream, and butter, is advised. Better options for your heart are fats derived from plants.

Ideas for Changing Your Diet in a Healthy Way

When it comes to eating well, small adjustments can have a tremendous impact. Think about substituting some of the meals you typically eat. For instance:

- Go for whole oranges rather than orange juice.
- Instead of white spaghetti or bread, try whole wheat versions.
- Add chopped vegetables to baked goods, soups, and casseroles. You might have to select softer vegetables that are simpler to chew as you become older.
- To cut back on salt, buy low-sodium soups and sauces or create your own.

- For your protein, choose lean meat cuts like skinless chicken breast or fish, or consider soy, legumes, or nuts as alternatives to meat.
- Substitute soft drinks and other sugary drinks with unsweetened sparkling water, milk, or yogurt instead.

Healthy Eating Choices

Choosing wise food selections is an excellent method to maintain a healthy diet. By adopting some of these behaviors, you can also enhance your nutrition.

Foods may lose part of their flavor as you become older, and some medications can alter how food tastes. To counteract this alteration, you can improve the flavor of your food by using spices and herbs rather than salt. Furthermore, salt-free spice combinations are available at stores.

Apply caution when deciding on a diet supplement. The greatest approach to receiving the nutrients you need is typically through food. If you need additional vitamins, tablets, or powders to supplement your diet, your doctor will be able to tell you.

Healthy eating includes drinking plenty of water. Drink plenty of water since as you become older, your sensation of thirst may diminish somewhat.

Make sure you have a color on your plate. In addition to making your food more appealing, including colored fruits and vegetables frequently increase its nutritious content.

Further Reminder.

Before making any significant dietary changes, consult your physician or a certified dietitian (RD). Your doctor can advise you on whether or not to include vitamins or other supplements in your daily diet and may propose specific modifications based on your health and the drugs you are taking.

CHAPTER FIVE

LIFESTYLE TO PROMOTE LONGEVITY.

The definition of longevity is "long life" or "a long duration of life." The word longaevitās is Latin in origin. You can see how the terms longus (long) and aevum (age) mix to form an idea in this word that refers to a person who lives a long period.

This definition's comparative character is its most crucial component. The average lifetime is the item that is implied by the phrase "long life."

Longevity is frequently defined by biologists as the typical lifespan anticipated under perfect circumstances. It's challenging to define such perfect circumstances. Many studies in medicine are being done to determine the "correct" kind and amount of exercise you should do, the ideal diet to follow, and whether or not specific medications or dietary supplements can lengthen your life.

Throughout the past century or so, there has been a fairly significant increase in life expectancy, largely as a result of medical advancements that have almost completely eradicated some lethal infectious diseases.

The average lifespan of a newborn born in 1900 was around 50 years. Currently, the average life expectancy in the United States is close to 79 years—81 years for women and 76 years for men—and in some other nations, it is even longer.

Humans will likely live far longer than we currently think. If people can establish the right habits of a good diet and exercise, people may live longer.

What Determines How Long You Live?

You might believe that your genes control how long you live, but in reality, genetics only contribute up to 25% to 30% of life expectancy. Your actions, attitudes, surroundings, and a small amount of luck account for the remaining factors. You may have heard about several methods for extending your life. Bear in mind that none of them have been demonstrated in people and that the majority are merely theories. Maintaining good health is the only way to extend your life.

LONGEVITY: 7 Healthy Practices That Would Make You Live Longer

For thousands of years, stories of endless youth and immortality have been passed down from generation to generation. The desire to live forever has been explored extensively throughout history, from ancient Greek mythology to modern literature and films. Although the Fountain of Youth may still only be a myth, due to advancements in science, medicine, and public health, it is now possible to live a longer life. Contrary to popular belief, however, a good lifestyle and habits rather than a supernatural cure are the secret to a long life.

It has been discovered that those who have lived the longest – into their nineties and hundreds — have comparable healthy practices, such as quitting smoking and maintaining a healthy weight, which reduce their risk of developing age-related chronic diseases including heart disease, cancer, and diabetes.

While aging is unavoidable, making healthy lifestyle adjustments today can help you age properly and perhaps extend your life by a few years. There are several things that can be done to promote longevity and in better health:

1. Keep moving.

It should come as no surprise that exercise benefits the body. But frequent physical activity, even in tiny doses, can not only keep you healthy and strong but also lengthen your life.

Exercise has been found to increase life expectancy, build bones and muscles, and lower the risk of age-related diseases like heart disease, high blood sugar, stroke, and several malignancies. In the meanwhile, research has connected sedentary habits and inactivity to a higher chance of dying young. According to one study, engaging in only 15 minutes of exercise or any physical activity each day can add three years to your life expectancy. Exercise can delay and even reverse cellular aging, according to research.

2. Give up smoking.
Smoking is linked to disease in almost every organ of the body and is the number one preventable cause of death in the United States. Smokers experience three times the mortality rate of non-smokers and pass away on average roughly 10 years earlier. Hence, giving up is never too late. Stopping smoking can extend your life by up to ten years and decrease the likelihood of heart attack, cardiovascular disease, stroke, respiratory cancer, and other cancers as well as other diseases. Therefore, the earlier you resign, the

better! It has been discovered that quitting smoking before age 40 reduces the chance of death from smoking-related diseases by 90%.

3. Drink moderately.

Overindulging in alcohol can increase your risk of getting heart disease, liver disease, high blood pressure, and some types of cancer, all of which can shorten your life expectancy. An adult's life expectancy may be reduced by one to two years if they drink 14 to 25 drinks per week, and by four to five years if they consume more than 25 drinks, according to one study. If you do drink, it's important to do so moderately—one drink for women per day, and up to two for men—to reduce these harmful effects on your health. According to several studies, consuming wine in particular (light to moderate) may even lower your chance of developing heart disease or stroke.

4. Reduce Your Stress Level.

Although stress is an inevitable part of life, excessive anxiety and worry can harm the body and interfere with practically all of its functions.

According to research, long-term stress can shorten life expectancy and raise the risk of high blood pressure, obesity, depression, and anxiety disorders. For instance, a Finnish study found that high levels of stress significantly shortened both men's and women's lives by more than two years. Fortunately, there are several techniques to control stress and safeguard your mental health, from writing, yoga, counseling, and meditation. You can even pick up certain hobbies like painting, learning an instrument, or knitting.

5. Foster Quality Relationships.

Relationships and friendships are good for your physical well-being in addition to being emotionally rewarding. According to a clinical evaluation of over 150 research, those with good social connections typically have a 50% higher probability of surviving than those with weaker social connections. The study discovered that the health risk of social isolation, alienation, or loneliness is greater than that of obesity or inactivity and is comparable to smoking 15 cigarettes per day. Strong, fulfilling relationships can lower stress and enhance general health while boosting emotions of happiness and life satisfaction.

6. Get proper sleep.

A consistent sleep pattern is also essential for the proper operation of your body. Many studies have demonstrated the connection between poor sleep and major health issues such as hypertension, inflammation, cardiovascular disease, and obesity, all of which shorten life expectancy. On the other hand, getting too much sleep has also been linked to a higher risk of heart disease and stroke, which can be detrimental to your health. A consistent sleeping plan every night, at least 7 to 8 hours of sleep can increase your longevity. Not getting enough sleep has some detrimental cognitive effects as it greatly affects the proper functioning of the brain. Therefore, it is of high importance that you get enough quality sleep.

7. Maintain a Balanced Diet.

We do not even need to delve too much into this one. Many people frequently consider their diet in terms of their immediate health objectives, such as weight loss or improved digestion. But, the food you consume today could have a significant long-term impact on your life, including how long you may live. It has been demonstrated that a balanced diet high in fruits, vegetables, fiber, and whole foods can help prevent inflammation and chronic diseases that account for the majority of early deaths, including diabetes, obesity, heart disease, hypertension, and some types of cancer.